Contents

Intro

Chapter One - The first time inside.

Chapter Two - Back to school.

Chapter Three - I don't need this shit anymore.

Chapter Four - Gartnavel adolescent unit

Chapter Five - Gartnavel part two

Chapter Six - An adult in an adult ward

Chapter Seven - The two-year break

Chapter 8- Caged voluntary

Chapter Nine - On the right direction home

Chapter Ten - Football brought me back

Chapter Eleven - Finding my wife

Chapter Twelve - Proper routine

Chapter Thirteen - The dream

Chapter Fourteen – Starting a family

Chapter Fifteen - The time to start writing

Chapter Sixteen - My thoughts

Chapter Seventeen - Doctors notes

Chapter Eighteen - Family thoughts

Chapter Nineteen - The St Andrews day interview

Chapter Twenty - The penultimate hope

The final chapter

Intro

Five guys were forcing me face down against the rugged carpet. I could see grit and stains in each groove. The veins in my neck were popping from all the shouting I was doing. I could feel the needle injecting me in the ass with drugs to sedate me. All whilst screaming for help!

I watched as my dad broke down and said "it would be ok" as I was pushed through the double doors, then into the room that I would call home.

I was a Sixteen-year-old skinny boy who had never been in a serious fight in his life.

This was the beginning of the fight against my own mind.

Monday the 4th of February 2002 my life came to an abrupt halt.

Throughout this book I will take you on a journey of my bi-polar (manic depression as first diagnosed) experience.

I will explain what it was like at each end of the bi-polar spectrum during my most difficult episodes. I will try and portray my state of mind at the time was and try and paint you a picture of what it was like living through it.

I have manged to build this story from obtaining doctors notes and recalling my own memories. Playing music from those years seems to trigger memories and I found that useful for what you are about to read.

My character pre diagnosis

Growing up in the years before 2002 I was always shy at school. It wasn't like I was stuck for words. It was like a restrained shyness. I just never had the confidence to project all my thoughts to people I didn't know very well.

It would be a different case with my close friends and family. I was more relaxed with them. I had confidence around them and wasn't afraid to express myself.

The first episode.

The weeks leading up to that point in my life were tough. My first proper relationship had broken down. My friends were starting to drift away from me, and I was putting too much pressure on myself to do well in school.

The trigger point happened when I stayed up all night lifting weights. My grandma was watching over me and couldn't hear the constant crashing of the weights colliding against the floor and the bench. I was relentless with the weights. I seemed to have bags of energy stored up to keep going. The truth was that my mind was racing, and it didn't give me time to focus on how tired I was. For that whole night I didn't have one ounce of sleep.

While I was working out, thoughts were playing over and over in my mind that I had to look great to be better than anyone else. I had to make myself look the best shape possible. Nobody was going to come close to me.

By the time Monday morning came I was so pumped up. It felt like my eyeballs were bursting out.

It was a crisp and fresh winters morning. But inside my thoughts were going at 100mph. One thought lead to an explosion of other thoughts each going in different directions.

I got myself into an argument with one of the boys I had always respected. He was captain of my primary school football team, popular and always had that great air of self-confidence about him.

My cousin had heard the commotion that I had created around myself and quickly took my arm and lead me away from the situation.

As I walked past a teacher at the RE base, she claimed that I must be on steroids!

The head teacher at the time was Mr King. He handled my situation brilliantly. He advised me that I had no option but to go home. He stated that other teachers had noticed a drastic change in me. I told him I was just trying show my true self. Maybe I was trying to be someone I always wanted to be.

Mr King drove me home and I could tell he was worried.

My parents had been informed of what had happened at school.

At the house my mum and dad were waiting for me. I was standing in the living room of the family home when I switched on teletext (for those of a younger age, it's basically Sky sports news but just text on a black screen). I would always look at this first thing in the morning. It was routine, just like reading the morning paper or engaging in social media feeds today.

I went straight to the sports section.

I noticed the top header of Hammy ski champion. That was my nickname at school, which has never left me. What did that mean?! Was it my first psychotic thought?

I started to trip out a bit, thinking that people were talking about me. I asked my mum to take a picture of that header on the tv just to prove I wasn't dreaming.

My parents immediately took me to my local doctors.

My dad had some words with my GP while I was sat in the waiting area. Just as soon as we had arrived, we left, and I jumped into my dad's car again. I pleaded with my dad just to take me back to school.

We set off and started to drive towards Paisley. I had thought that he was simply taking me to his work for me to calm down.

We drove past Kersland, my sister's old school and on to a part of Paisley that I was unfamiliar with.

As soon as I saw the sign "Dykebar" that's when I really started to panic.

I had heard about that place at school. The nuthouse!

This could not be happening to me. I wasn't crazy!

We walked into the old acute building. Ward one B to be exact. The building was very dated and looked like something out of a horror film.

The long corridor with rooms on either side lead to a fire exit at the end. This fire exit door at the very end had a glass panel where the sun would rise, giving the look of some light at the end of the tunnel.

Unfortunately, the ward felt dark, and my lights were about to be switched off.

To begin with I was left outside waiting at one of the small interview rooms. These were situated just at the main entrance of the ward. I was stuck waiting for my dad to finish speaking with a doctor.

This seemed like an eternity, waiting on someone else to decide on my fate without me even being involved.

This set the standard, the standard of my involvement of my OWN mental health in the years to come. Doctors keeping me out of the loop. Only communicating with my parents with stuff that really mattered.

How do you think that effects someone's state of mind being shut out? Not being allowed to give my version of the events or participate in the plans for my development.

I was called into a room with my dad. The doctor placed a cup of water on the table along with a blue pill in a shot glass next to it. The doctor advised me to take the pill. I was told it would help. Help what?!

I didn't believe in taking pills to get better. I would rather ride out any illness and fight it on my own without any intervention. Who knows what could be in that pill anyway?

I thought back to an old film I had seen. The matrix. The main character Neo was offered the red or blue pill. One of the pills would take him out his reality.

I drank the water and used the bottom of the empty glass to smash the pill up on the table. Not a chance in hell was I taking that.

It's at that point I was given my marching orders. The heavies appeared, and the double doors to the ward opened to close off my world as I knew it.

Chapter one - The first time inside.

"Walking down corridors like the walking dead,

No energy to break bread or even lift my head.

With my mind in a daze, all that I see is haze,

I am struggling to face these days,

But they are telling me it's just a faze."

Rewind to the moment I was brought inside that room kicking and screaming from my lungs.

The dust had settled, and the medication had kicked in. I was alone in that tiny room. Suddenly my loud outburst was drowned out by other patients.

This was an adult ward and there were plenty of others who could shout louder and longer than me.

As I sat on the bed and looked out of the window, I could hear screams and moans coming from other rooms. A guy was pacing the corridor with his steel toe capped boots on. His stomps smashed against the floor with each over exaggerated step.

I was terrified, my door wasn't locked, and I thought at any moment someone was going to burst through that door. (not knowing it would be a member of staff)

After a few hours (which seemed like days) went by I was asked by one of the nurses if I wanted toast. She took me down and sat me in a chair at the nurse's desk. A few of the older nurses gasped when they saw how young I was.

I will always remember a nurse named Sandra looking deep into my eyes and saying, "we won't keep you here any longer than we need to".

After getting toast I was free to walk about the ward and mix in the different lounge areas. One room was a smoking room, this was the place the older inpatients spent most of their time.

As soon as the door opened to that room, you could see a cloud of smoking circling around the ceiling. Together with the unpleasant smell of smoke it had a damp smell to go with it.

It was in this room the next day where I had my first "major" psychotic thought. Rangers were playing Celtic and it was live on tv. I thought I was able to control the players movement in my mind, much like playing a FIFA computer game with a controller. I genuinely felt I made Bert Konterman's score that wonder goal.

Later, in that first night as darkness crept in, I made my mind up to get out. A button at the end of the corridor marked "exit" this was the obvious escape.

I pressed the button and pushed the door open. I was immediately out at the main entrance. I pushed the final door open and I was out, but I had no idea where to go. I ran into the field directly behind the main building to keep out of sight. However, I was closely followed by the on-rushing staff.

At this point I was still on a high and my energy levels were still good, even after the sedation injections. I sidestepped a few lunges and danced through other advances. But, in the end I was rugby tackled to the ground and then lifted by my arms and legs back into my room.

This attempted escape must have been rubber stamped in my notes for everyone to see.

I was prescribed a drug called olanzapine and was told that I must take this. I would get home sooner by taking they said. Anything to get out of this hell hole I thought.

This medication was far too easy to go down as it melted on my tongue.

The side effects were like nothing I had experienced in my short life up to then. I was constantly hungry, and my thought process was clouded.

I found it hard to focus or keep my eyes away from looking at the floor.

My vision was distorted, much like tunnel vision and I started to feel tired all the time. My balance was all over the place. I felt like I was on a boat at sea when I stood up.

I guess my tiredness was a mixture of the medication kicking in and the start of the come down from the high of the manic episode. This was also coupled with the lack of sleep and of course my mind working on an emergency back-up mode after being burned out.

It's not hard to see the reasons why I started to balloon up. The amount of food being consumed together with the lack of movement was starting to show.

One of the main memories I have from that period was when my sister with down syndrome visited. I gave her a drink from my sink, a mixture of cold and hot water. This was "a cure" for her, a fucking cure for down syndrome, what the hell was I thinking of??!

Throughout my life I had become very protective of my sister. Growing up she was just my sister and I looked at her no different to my other sister.

However, when I was out of the house with her, I could see how most people would react to her. The looks she got would break me every time. On a few occasions, after some sniggering out loud by other people, I would want to go and fight with whoever did it. I would never want to show my sister how it affected me, so I would just walk on and leave it.

The times I walked on I would always regret I didn't say anything. Half of the time those people would have just been plain ignorant to her condition. The others would just be showing off to their friends.

One day I was getting the bus to school. This bus stopped outside my house at the same time my sisters bus picked her up.

A few boys at the back of the bus started to mock her. I kept my mouth shut throughout the whole 2-mile journey but when I was in the school grounds, I couldn't hold back any longer. I approached the main instigator of the chat and called him out straight away. I gave him the look where I would have immediately knocked him to the floor. The guy backed down and he never behaved like that in my presence again.

The other main memory which still bugs me was one of the male staff members.

He was a heavy-set guy with short hair and a bushy beard. On one occasion as I was looking out my door window when he walked past. I got a fright and launched my bottle of Lucozade into the air. He then barged in, griped my thumb in a lock behind my back and started to twist. I felt some excruciating pain and tried to get loose. In doing so he held on tighter and pushed his knees on my legs. I was sure my wrist had snapped.

Looking back, not at one point did he call for any assistance. And I knew he liked the pain he inflicted on me. The look on his face was pure evil.

If I was his build and age would he have done that to me?

Cutting back to the story, during this episode I was hypomanic. My confidence was sky high. It's the best feeling in the world. This huge self believe is something that I craved to get back ever since.

I could turn my hand to anything, my great passion of football was now the simplest thing I could do. I could see the game so simply. I knew exactly how I could achieve my dream. I am naturally two footed. I was going to be a legend. I appeared to have this great self-belief in myself and believed that was what I was previously missing to perform. I believed I could excel on a world stage.

One of the main tell-tale signs of bipolar is grandiose ideas or flights of fancy. Was my idea of becoming a professional footballer a grandiose idea? Was it so impossible to achieve? Or was this the correct frame of mind to become an elite player?

Monday 4th February 2002-

Wednesday 27th February 2002

23 days in total spent in hospital

Age 16

Medication: Olanzapine

I feel the rain on my skin, as I stand on the inside looking out.

This pain hurts my brain when the tablets kick out.

The envy of passers-by freely walking about.

Time ticking by with my feet nowhere near the ground.

I am lost in here, and I'm never going to be found.

Those profound thoughts slowly being downed.

Another dose of medication with a shot glass on the tray.

Again...

Again...

Again, my heart's slipping away.

Will someone please take me away.

I've had too much. Please don't make me stay.

Medication again... when will this stop.

The hour hand has jumped and fallen from the clock.

When will this stop?

Chapter two- Back to school.

Words can't describe how nervous I was on the first morning going back into school. I knew I had to get the first day out the way. After spending 23 days in a mental hospital I wanted to forget that experience very quickly and get back to "normal" life.

I knew that someone would have said where I had been and by now everyone would have known. These things spread like wildfire especially at schools.

My biggest fear was coming back to school. With all the stigma attached to someone who was "Mental".

I was worried what people would think of me. Would my school friends treat me differently than before?

Would they mock and goad me for being unwell?

The moment arrived for me to walk through the school gates.

The walk up-hill seemed extremely daunting going up to the school building. This was a huge step for me. Whilst walking along the tech corridor I saw pupils double taking at me. Without saying a word, I made my way through to the back area where I would usually meet my friends before registration.

Before I could catch a breath, the bell rang to go to registration.

That was me. I was back and I just tried to keep my head down.

But at that point I was over self-stigmatising what people thought of me.

At the time, I was the type of person who cared what people thought of me, maybe that's why I was shy around people that I didn't know very well. I wouldn't want to make a fool of myself and be ridiculed for it.

Looking back, I shouldn't have cared what others thought. But as a kid in that situation this was going to be harder than facing up to the illness itself.

Outside of school I was always at my happiest with the group of friends I had whilst growing up. I wasn't shy around them and I never thought about what they would think of me.

Self-pressure

I always thought I should aim for the best academically.

Generally, at the time I was more practical than academical.

Rory's raps song

One of my friends was experimenting with his music and had written a rap that included me in it.

I still remember the words to this day. Even-though I only heard it once. I remember those lines clearly.

"mate locked in Dykebar, man I'm feeling you.

Fell my presence so called adolescent

Manic depressive, teach yourself some happy lessons"

What would my happy lessons be?

Chapter Three - I don't need this shit anymore.

School had settled down and everything seemed to be back to 'normal'.

Naturally, in my eyes that if everything was back to normal, medication wouldn't be needed.

I moved bi-polar to the back of my mind. So far back it was almost out of sight.

In addition, I hated what I saw in the mirror. The boy staring back wasn't me. My belly was getting huge. I blamed it on the medication.

This was the moment I started to self-medicate.

To start, I would skip a night's dose, this followed by two nights until I had missed a full week.

I was starting to feel less tired. I spent less time in bed. When late nights started to coincide by the early rises, and I felt like my thoughts started to run clearer.

In truth I was losing control. The problem with mania in bipolar is when it starts to grip, it's the best feeling in the world to experience. I never stopped to think why I was feeling so good. Why would anyone question having an elated state of mind?

Family close to me would start to see the subtle differences in me that I wouldn't have recognised, and in all honesty wouldn't want to. I would have given anything to feel like that again, the on top of the world feeling was creeping back in and I was loving it.

Chapter Four - Gartnavel adolescent unit

The 2nd episode

The build up to this episode may have seemed like any other teenage problem, rebelling against my parent's authority.

However, the moment I was locked in my house unable to leave I knew this would become a tipping point.

Being forced to remain in one place never sits well with me. It gives me cabin fever, and with bipolar those feelings become intensified.

An ambulance was called when I started to literally bounce off walls to get out.

Instead of spending time in Dykebar I was transferred to Gartnavel adolescent unit as they finally had a spare bed for me.

Not for one moment could I have imagined the length of time I would need to spend in there.

The T-shaped unit was locked with a key from the inside, instead of those helpful buttoned exits.

No escaping this place. Unless it's out a broken window or through the unlocked doors.

The rubber stamp from my notes must have been in full force in this unit. I was given no fresh air and couldn't even get out with supervised time. This effectively made it a prison for me and would lead to greater strain and mental anguish.

I remember having a conversation with one of the staff members in the ward saying that he was faster than me, and if I did try to escape from the unit, he would catch me. He was a cocky wee bastard if I remember right.

The first week and a half was spent like a caged animal. No fresh air or any room to exercise.

Being confined to one room with only my own thoughts to occupy my mind was a head fuck.

Looking back on the doctor's notes it clearly shows how I was being kept in a room and then held against my will in the adolescent unit which I feel affected me more than the actual illness. The aggression I was displaying was intensifying with every moment locked in there.

If someone had taken the time to get to know my interests, what I did outside school, my hobbies and what makes me happy, maybe just maybe a quicker recovery would have happened.

I had no means to blow off any physical energy which would then come across as reckless behaviour and aggression.

During most weekends I would gaze out of my bedroom window and stare at the guys playing football at the bottom of the grass hill. Longing so desperately just to be involved.

One day, I wrote a "help me" note with toothpaste on the window. This could be read clearly from the other side. I wanted out that desperately.

However, with no help coming any time soon and a visitor to the unit pointing out the message to staff I was made to clean it off.

On the flip side to this unit, some there was some genuine staff that were very good with me. Jen, Robert and Chris notably helped me immensely.

I was prescribed lithium, the mood stabiliser, to take. I initially struggled with lithium as I had to give blood frequently. The blood tests checked that the levels were correct in my system.

On the first occasion my eldest sister joined me in the doctor's room to get the first drop of blood out of my veins. In my head I didn't want this to be the norm, having to go out of my way to check blood levels for the correct dosage of medication. Eventually the notion of this and the fear of strangers putting a needle into my arm disappeared. I suppose with three tattoos to date prove I have overcome that fear.

Weekly meetings were held with doctors. I felt that there had to be some level of trust with doctors. How can I be expected to speak to a random person openly about what's going on in my head?

I struggled with this sort of communication. And often refused to speak.

Most of the time is was again waiting on the outside of meetings and not getting the chance to say my side. When I got my five mins to shine, I was unable to find the words to describe how I felt. This led to more time spent in hospital. Although I was a child, I never recall any doctors sitting down with me and getting my thoughts on what was happening. Opinions always came from other sources.

Well apart from being given a short booklet on Manic Depression, that seemed to be my only real insight to what was going on.

I wasn't told about the daily struggle, what signs to watch for and stuff I really needed to know.

I sometimes wonder. How would someone with no mental health issues react to being locked in a unit and not demand to leave the place they are being kept.

Was there a stage where I was on a level playing field mentally and then being told I would have to spend more time in hospital. Did this have a detrimental effect on me?

In hindsight I should have kept all my thoughts down on paper and presented them to the doctors at each meeting.

Friday 10th May 2002 -

Wednesday 18th Sept 2002

131 days in total

Age 16/17

Medication Lithium

Chapter Five - Gartnavel part two

Third episode

My first part time job was in JJB Sports. This is was the scene of my first hallucination. I managed to convince myself that the shops radio loudspeaker was talking about me. That caused me to break down in tears in-front of a customer.

The shift was a blur and as it finished, I looked up and saw all the staff at the back wall. They were huddled in a group. I was standing alone down at the front of the store.

In my mind they were all plotting against me.

That night I had to leave the family house and took my dog up to my aunt and uncles house.

I didn't want to stay with my mum and dad, I needed to be in a different environment.

I slept on the couch at my aunt and uncles with my uncle sleeping on the opposite couch keeping an eye on me.

I always held my uncle in high regard and for him to watch over me calm me down made me feel safe.

Outside of their front living room window was a hill in the distance with random trees clustered together. When I was young, I always thought they looked like an army of soldiers.

This is when everything started to go weird. I looked out the window during the night and saw loads of different colours up on the hill.

My mind was playing tricks on me and whenever I closed my eyes, I could see flashes of bright colours. I needed help!

The following morning, I was picked up by my mum and dad along with the dog. We drove home and parked in the driveway. I put one foot out of the car to set myself, the second step was full on sprint down the driveway and away from the house. I didn't know where I was going to run to until I heard a voice calling my name. A familiar voice, the one voice that I listened to. It was my cousin. She was driving past the cycle track while I was sprinting up the hill. She sounded knackered while telling me to slow down because I was running too fast.

I listened to everything she told me. But I still needed some sort of release from my thoughts.

What was happening to me? I was tripping out, a lack of sleep, and my thoughts were racing again. I had lost contact with reality. I started to believe people weren't who they were.

The Truman effect

For anyone who hasn't seen the Truman show, the leading character (played by Jim Carrey) is born into a tv show. The life he lives is 24/7 in front of a live tv audience and his whole world is manufactured around him.

Before I knew, I was back in Gartnavel. I had a room to myself with constant supervision, but it was just me and my thoughts, I started to believe the Truman effect was happening to me. Whilst in this head space, complied with no fresh air and the beginnings of being institutionalised, my thoughts had drifted to points where I questioned everything. I questioned my life, my family, my whole existence and even live itself.

Why was this happening to me? What sort of twisted experiment was I part of?

The reason in my head was obvious. The Truman show must be about me. I firmly believed everyone in the hospital were actors! Those actors being hospital staff, patients and then when my family came up to visit, I believed they actors too. Any rational thoughts were gone at that moment.

At one point I was advised to go for a shower to freshen up. That's it I thought, this was going to be the big reveal. They were finally going to tell me about the tv show I was the star of.

I remember taking some time in the shower, composing myself.

I went into the shower thinking I was the messiah.

Then I emerged from the shower with a smile on my face. Quickly, that was wiped away and I realised nothing had changed. I was told to go straight back to my room.

Wait, I wasn't the messiah?! Turns out I was just a very naughty boy! And probably stinking to! I had neglected the daily routine that I would normally do at home.

It took me a good few days to snap out of this state. Maybe the medication was working. Or the high was starting to come down naturally.

During that time, I had stopped taking the medication the staff were giving me. I thought the drugs would stop me from knowing "the truth". I would put the tablets in my mouth on one side, and as I drank the small shot of water, I would spit the tablet into my finger which held the cup. As I gave the shot cup back, they would look in my mouth to see the tablet gone. I would proceed to shove it behind my back and then dispose of it later.

And they thought I was daft?!

So, back at Gartnavel again, I had barely been away from the place. Some of the familiar faces were still in.

Danielle

One of the girls I had met in the unit was someone who had the same sort of issues as me. In Danielle's case she was strongly opposed to authority figures but wanted to be popular with her peers.

She understood me and left a lasting impression with me. Her thoughts were deep and meaningful, and I understood her methods of thinking.

Years later I had heard terrible news about her. Trying to be popular with her peers made her take risks that she shouldn't have. One of those risks ended up being her last. I hope she found peace in all her darkest moments.

Whilst still in hospital I still aspired to sit my higher exams. Mr King my head teacher from school remained in close contact. He was genuinely sincere in how he spoke to me. You can tell from a person by the way they look at you, making eye contact if they are being serious or not.

He had offered me the chance to repeat 6th year at school and get my qualifications that way.

For me to drop down a year and have no friends was one of the main reasons I declined.

The embarrassment of repeating the year with guys the year below me was a definite no go for me.

The main reason was of course my state of mind and wanting to take it slowly this time.

Being in the unit, one way for me to combat my boredom was to eat. I started to sink lower and accepted my fate that I would in the hospital for a prolonged period.

But then when I accepted that I would need to stay longer, did that show a depressed state? Thus, keeping me in even longer?

That dream of waking up at home and it's all been a nightmare, then actually waking up and having to coming to terms that I am still locked away.

Eventually I would start to get day passes home. These were step by step and then started to include overnight stays home. The sense of relief when allowed to go home a day at a time was unreal.

Sunday 27th November 2002- Tuesday 15th April 2003

139 days in total

Age 17

Medication Amisulpride

Chapter Six - An adult in an adult ward

4th episode

Saturday the 15th of November 2003 Scotland 1-0 Holland

A deflected James McFadden goal sent the tartan army into raptures. My Dad and I had our arms round each other as we celebrated.

The elation of that night with my dad, brother in law and his dad at Hampden was the celebration before the heartbreak.

The high that I was experiencing was starting to manifest into a full on bipolar high.

The warning signs were there but I chose to overlook them.

To start with I bought an 8k car and took out a grand loan to pay for Christmas presents. From the grand loan I managed to squander away £750 within an hour.

I booked a holiday for around 6 friends and I was going to pay for it all.

Bearing in mind I didn't have a job to fund these repayments.

All of these were triggers I didn't take notice of.

That reckless money spending was a major trigger. If I had the disposable income to afford it, that would be no problem. In my head I was getting a job yesterday to pay for it all.

The morning of Wednesday 19th November 2003 I had dressed in suit with a training top under my shirt.

The training shirt was a St. Mirren training top which I had bought while doing voluntary coaching at Love Street.

I left the house armed with my football folder. This was filled with autographs, match programmes, ticket stubs and my ideas/philosophy for how I thought football should be played.

I arrived at Love Street to speak to the head of youth development, David Longwell, who was my main point of contact while gaining voluntary experience. I wanted to demonstrate to him how much I wanted a job after already taking part in voluntary sessions at the club. I hoped to show him how much I loved football and why I would have been a great member of staff.

I felt if I was involved in coaching and around the club, I would be noticed and hopefully I would be able to work my way up to play for the club.

When I went to speak to David, he informed me that police were looking for me.

My nose started to bleed, and my heart sank. Yes, I had be acting strange recently but surely this must have been a huge misunderstanding.

I couldn't stem the flow of blood. I glanced out of David's glass windowed office and saw two policemen walk in. I kept my head down trying not to be noticed. This made the drip worse.

David asked me if I was ok and to talk to him, I couldn't bring myself to tell him what was really going on with me. No way could I explain to him (who I had high admiration of) about my deep underlining issues.

The two policemen came in and grabbed my upper arms to escort me out of the building. I had a quick look back over my shoulder where I could see everyone looking at me. "That's that fucked" I thought to myself.

The policemen still had a tight grip round my arms, which was evident with the deep bruising days later when my friends came to visit.

Was it necessary for them to do that? I relaxed my body a bit and felt them clutching tighter.

I wasn't a criminal or kicking off with them to merit those actions on me.

The officers initially drove me to the RAH. However, when I was asked to sit in a wheelchair to go down to be assessed in the ward, I point blank refused. They wanted to put me in a fucking wheelchair! Why?!

Is mental ill health a physical injury that prevents me from walking??

After that refusal I was then put back in the police car to be assessed in Dykebar.

The policemen then began to discuss how to get to Dykebar to which I butted in by saying I would give them directions……how long have you been on for? What time do you finish at?...

As the new taxi drivers dropped me off at the recently built acute east ward building my life was about to come crashing down, much like Scotland's second leg payoff defeat in Holland.

So, there I was, back at the Mental health hospital and yes you guessed it I was waiting outside of a room while a doctor gathered information on my "well-being".

What seemed like hours passed by and then as quick as a lightning bolt I was told I was being sectioned.

I was given the room next to the nurse's station and put on constant observation.

A couple of familiar nurses appeared and gave me the low down.

Sandra, Dougie and Sheena were some friendly faces I remembered.

On one occasion I remember having a full-blown argument with my Dad. The nurse's station was shaped like the front of a court room and I was the judge. I remember at the time I felt like I was looking down on this happening, the words quickly flowing off my tongue, they were being blurted out with no thoughts or control over them.

Unlike the previous admission, after a few days I felt like I could have conversations with fellow in-patients.

After all I was now an adult in an adult ward, I felt more relaxed in exchanging conversations with people that were in with me.

I was amazed at the wide spectrum of people's background that had been admitted alongside me.

From Doctors, ex policemen, teachers, father's, husband's and people with recurring issues.

One of the boys my age, Paul, and I developed a great bond.

He had very similar interests as me. From his music tastes to his youth spent at the boy's brigade.

We would spend hours in the music room chilling out with our favourite music which happened to be hip-hop at the time. From American stars such as Kanye West then me introducing Paul to homegrown Scottish rappers in Loki and Blackheart.

He would show off his dance moves and we would imagine being out at night clubs performing them. This was a far cry from the reality we were in.

Paul had told me of his failed attempt at the Erskine bridge, it was always in the back of my mind about his safety.

When walking in and around the ward I noticed other patients with wrist supports and asked one lady how she come about the injury.

The girl said it was due to a heavy restraint she received from a certain member of staff. Funnily enough it was the same member of staff who gave me a huge grin before restraining me by himself in my room away back at my very first admission.

How many other people did his grip snap tendons and break bones in his apparent role of care?

Wednesday 19th November 2003 -

Tuesday 27th Jan 2004

69 days in total

Age 18

Medication quetiapine

All the times that we had spent,

Under the same roof not paying any rent.

You were like a brother to me,

One apple falling not far from the tree.

You took matters into your own hands,

And stopped a future wearing the same brands.

If I could rewind time. And commit one crime.

I would break down that wall and made sure you didn't fall.

Rest easy Paul.

Chapter Seven - The two-year break

28th Jan 2004 to 21st December 2005

Hypersensitivity

Coming out of hospital after being institutionalised was difficult at the best of times. After Gartnavel all my senses seemed to be heightened. The smallest sound around me would explode like a firework set off in my ears. My environment seemed new. It was like being born again and opening my eyes to this huge world in front of me.

I had always loved the buzz of the town at peak times during the day and night. However, seeing so many people at once after very little was frightening. I would normally skip through the crowds, managing not to bump into anyone. During that time, I just seemed to get in everyone's way, which would just add to my feelings of worthlessness and deepened my low mood.

Meeting my friends socially in the city centre's pubs and clubs was so difficult. I couldn't have face to face conversations with my friends. This was due to the fact I couldn't tune into their words. I was being drawn away by background noise around me. I could start to hear ringing sounds and at those points I would need to leave the situation.

I could never explain to my friends what was happening. Looking back, I fucking wish I did. Instead of thinking that I had to man up and just ignore what was happening. By acting like a man, I should have told my friends why I was acting weird, being open and honest to them would have been manning up.

My first objective when I left hospital was to get my provisional licence back and sit my driving test. I passed first time in May which was a huge step for me. The freedom to get up and go whenever I wanted.

My main goal when I left hospital was to make it my mission to chase my dream of playing professional football.

I sent letters and emails to all professional clubs within one hundred miles radius of my house and my favourite English premier league team Newcastle.

Newcastle was the only team who came back to me. They offered me a chance to go down and train in partnership with premier skills.

The weeks trial programme with premier skills was a great insight in what I had to do to become an elite footballer.

I was given the number 69 which I thought was symbolic as I had just finished 69 days in hospital. Could this be some sort of sign of great things to come.

However, it was obvious from the start the different fitness levels required to be at the top. The athletic guys weren't necessary the best footballers, but these guys excelled and excited the coaches and scouts watching on. Those guys would sprint pass defenders and chase runners within seconds.

Ultimately it wasn't my time and was told to come back next summer and go away to work on my fitness.

Coming back up the road I realised I had to be playing football regularly.

I looked in the local paper and found a local team in the Westend of Glasgow. Before one of teams training sessions, I arrived early and watched a session that was on before us.

I recognised one of the guys playing as I had met him whilst playing football on holiday. After this chance meeting we ended up starting a "bromance" playing football and pool every other day.

He invited me to play with his mates on a Sunday. The first time that I turned up, I quickly realised which grass park they played on. It was the spare grass area at the bottom of the adolescent unit. I real clarity moment for me.

I was finally on the other side of the glass to where I had spent so long looking out. I took five minutes in my car after the kickabout to take in this moment. So much clarity filled my head.

Come the summer of 2005 I was flying! I was on such I high. I had two weeks abroad with the boys for the first time. This was followed by a weekend at T in the park with school mates.

The T in the park weekend ended for me on the Sunday night by watching my favourite band Kasabian. I jumped on the first bus back home on the Sunday night to be ready to drive down the following morning for the next trail.

My body had taken a battering, but my mind was still racing.

Before I went on holiday the "great" idea I had was to be high as a kite for this trial, that would mean I would be ultra-confident with endless amounts of energy, and I would be able to showcase my full potential.

The trail began and as expected I was flying, smashing all the fitness tests and in charge of the ball.

As Tuesday morning hit, I had slept in, I could barely open my eyes and couldn't move my body, the come down from the high was like a sky dive, I had hit rock bottom over-night.

I couldn't believe it, I forced myself to get up and ready to head over to the briefing room which was in full flow. My legs were like jelly and I had the motion feeling again like I was on a boat.

I wanted to shut myself out, I wanted to chuck it there and then. How could I have been so naive to think that missing medication would have done me any good.

I managed to scrape my way through to the Friday but left before any feedback was given.

My dream was over! In my eyes at least. I was in no fit state mentally to drive myself on any further.

I packed my stuff and left. Eyes sunken on the floor.

On the drive back up the road I stopped at Gretna Green.

I parked up at a football pitch, took a ball out, put my boots on. I proceeded to kick the ball high into the sky several times, then on the final kick, booted the ball far into the opposite field. I was done. Game over!

At this point I was in a crossroads in my life. I had no idea what I wanted to do next. Football was all I had ever dreamed of doing.

A few months would pass by before I would find out what was in store for me.

Chapter 8 - Caged voluntary

Wednesday 21st December 2005

As Christmas was approaching, I was on high again, the medication I was taking seemed to have little or no effect anymore.

My world was about to take another nosedive.

Coming to terms with the realisation that I have a problem. A problem that had to be fixed. The realisation came to me suddenly in my mum and dads old house.

I was standing at the front door looking back down the hall. My CPN (community psychiatric nurse) was halfway down the hall with my mum and dad behind him at the living room doorway.

I was about to storm out of the house after my CPN had come to see me.

This meeting was called for from a family member who had been worried about me.

I used to always blame my family for going behind my back to seeking help for me. I guess they were only looking out for me. Maybe, too much help was a bad thing. The slightest thing that I did would have been scrutinised as being part of the so called, illness.

So back to my Cpn's appearance. The look he gave me told me what I already knew. He didn't have to say anything. I could see it in his eyes. The look told the story.

I knew I had to get help. I needed to face up to my "illness".

It was at that moment I admitted I had a problem. Although I never said it out loud to anyone, it hit me hard and resonated throughout me.

I made up my mind to go into Dykebar voluntary. My Cpn said he would drive me up. I felt safe around him, he was like that big brother figure I hadn't had. I suppose that just highlights how good he was at his job to be able to make me feel at ease during what was another stressful moment in my life.

Not long after I admitted myself into the adult ward, I found out that a Section was slapped over my head, again! I was livid. I had come in voluntary of my own accord. Fuck them! I had become so angry at that point, I wanted to leave, they just wanted to mess with my mind again. Cue the alarm bells buzzing from the belt packs strapped on to the members of staff, as my hulk face took over. When I kicked off, I would never hurt anyone, however the fixtures and fittings didn't feel any pain.

I had come in to fight my illness, now I felt like I had to fight the whole world again.

On top of being in hospital I knew along with the section being place on my head, my driving licence would have been suspended for at least 3 months from that point. You might think 3 months isn't a long time, a short time is always long time in young man's mind.

After spending Christmas in the ward, I found out I would still be in at Hogmanay.

As the countdown to the bells started, I went to my room alone. Radio One's Scott Mills was blaring from my phone. With ten minutes left to the bells and I ran myself a shower. As the year drew in, I jumped in the shower. I was fresh for the New year. A fresh mindset and a clear understanding to promise myself that I would never end up back inside these walls again.

Transfer to the Rah

After spending just over a month in that ward I was given the chance to go to the more familiar surroundings of the RAH, the hospital where I was born. The same place I went to fix a broken leg and wrist. You know, those physical injuries that people can see at face value.

A few days after arriving I was given time to go to the hospital physio room, or the small gym. That little bit of time to exercise was great.

I started to build up my time getting out of the ward. I would use this time to go jogging around the area.

The patients who were in with me were a great help too. Everyone with a common goal of overcoming their issues within a relatively short time scale.

For this period in hospital and every other period the constant by my side was my mum and dad. My mum came to see me twice a day without fail and my dad would try his best to do the same, but work prevented that.

.

However, with my family visiting me, it made it hard to stay in the hospital and not want to go home with them.

But I managed to get through it, it was fucking hard, I won't lie.

As the old saying goes. Fifth time's lucky eh? A total of 452 days had been notched up at that point in and around hospital care. That's 10,848 hours, surely, I've served my time by now.

Wednesday 21st December 2005 to Thursday 26th Jan 2006

Dykebar

Thursday 26 Jan 2006 to

Tuesday 21st March 2006

90 days in total

Age 20

Medication Depakote and Risperidone

Chapter Nine - On the right direction home

In my mind, going from Dykebar to the RAH was a huge step in the right direction.

The stigma of being in a mental hospital had been lifted, granted that I was in ward two for acute mental health.

Stigma was always something I used to be very self-conscious about.

I refused to disclose my bi-polar to people and would make up stories rather than tell people the truth about me.

A clear time of not telling the truth was when I was working "voluntary" at a sports centre where I was advised that I should have been getting paid.

Instead of me saying why I was working there and explaining I was taking part with support from a charity to help me get back into work, I simply said "yeah" I should be getting paid.

I would take the easy route out. Too ashamed to admit I had a mental health issue. Would they have looked down on me? Probably not, maybe they would have respected me more. I still couldn't face explaining what was wrong with me and why I was working voluntary.

I felt as a man I shouldn't show any sort of weakness.

The looking good factor

As a young man in my mind to attract the opposite sex I would need to look attractive physically. I would push my body to extreme conditions. That was never any good for my mental health. These "extreme" diets and exercise would involve little or no appetite, a lack of sleep and long-distance running. These runs would often be at full pelt. Or as fast as my current fitness would allow.

Over the years I have learned that to stay in a good mind frame I must have good rest days and try and get the minimum night sleep required to re-energise.

I know the saying of a healthy body equals a healthy mind. However, I know I can't push myself too far to achieve this perfect physical image or I will suffer from the manic side of bi-polar.

Canteen staff in Dykebar -v- same people at a night club in town

One night I remember queuing up at a Glasgow night club. Two girls who had served me in the canteen in Dykebar were standing in front of me in the queue. One of the girls had recognised me and began to ask where she recognised me from. She seemed to be interested in finding out where she knew me from. Before I could get the chance to revel the information, the other girl looked at me, she must have instantly known where and pulled her friend away before point blank ignoring me.

For someone to stop talking to me because of where I had been was extremely difficult for me to take in. It broke my confidence and from that point I knew I wasn't going to enjoy my night. I made an excuse and left half an hour later to go home alone.

I was still coming to terms with being back at home, I was anxious about going to my local pharmacy to collect medication.

It really bothered me seeing someone face to face to collect bipolar tablets. Years down the line that's not a problem, it was just my attitude back then.

The foundations of my life had been ripped up and I was slowly starting to find my feet again.

Continuing with the forward momentum was my CPN with his great support.

An A4 cheat sheet was created. This included signs to watch for. These consisted of irritability, increased talking, excessive exercise, lack of sleep, over thinking, overspending, rapid thoughts and increased social scene for mania. The depressive side of it would almost be the exact opposite thing of each item to watch for.

Chapter Ten - Football brought me back

The weeks after my final hospital spell my motivation and energy levels were at rock bottom.

I was stuck in a rut with nothing on the horizon.

A chance meeting with an old school mate (on one of the rare days that I made my way to a local shop) would change that rut completely.

He played for the local amateur football team and invited me to come along to training. This is when I started to gain back control mentally and physically.

I was the most unfit guy at my first training session, but I knew I had to push through it.

I was around the 15 stone mark, well overweight from my usual fighting weight of 12 stone 7.

The manager who I will be forever be grateful to must have seen something in me, because I think that if it was anyone else, he would have told me to beat it.

After about six weeks of hill sprints and the killer square I had lost 2 stones.

I felt amazing.

Rewind to six weeks earlier to the first session. I had gone straight back to bed and couldn't move.

The next morning and mornings that followed were tough to get out and about, but I had set my target for the next training session. A step at a time. Something to focus on.

Football was again my focal point in life.

Depression is not just feeling sad, and the no motivation factor, depression feels like your being strapped down with a heavy weight. Try all you want but nothing will get you up. Even if you find some amount of energy to sit up, the energy you have just used vanishes and you fall back down again.

The struggle is fucking real!

Fast-forward a few months and I am back! My friends are around me again, I have started a new job, I am doing well socially, physically and most importantly mentally.

Monday 7th April 2008 at 6.30pm. Ibrox stadium. The dream becomes a reality. I am playing football for Rangers. Number 8 on the left side of midfield. It might only be a charity game, but this is the moment I had dreamt of since I was knee high to a grasshopper.

It was only 45 mins of the first half in the game and it felt like 5 minutes, but it was the best thing that ever happened to me up to that point in my life.

Soccer circus

The new job that I had started came about after I asked to work for free at Kevin Keegan's Soccer Circus. The assistant manager said Free. No, you can have a job here".

To be accepted like that was a great feeling, and to work with one of my footballing hero's growing up was a chance in a lifetime.

Kevin Keegan's brand of football with Newcastle was one of the reasons I started following them.

The exciting football they produced from the likes of Faustino Asprilla to rocket finishes from Alan Shearer drew me in.

I was in there for about a year before sales started to decline and staff levels were cut. This was the best working time I had ever had. Playing football, coaching kids, and working with other people with the same interests as me, it was the dream job.

Chapter Eleven - Finding my wife

I met my wife at the perfect time.

I was a year into new 9-5 steady job and was mentally and physically stable.

She was attractive, witty and an unbelievable character. Words don't do justice.

It had been just under four years since I had left hospital for the last time. I'm sure if I had met her earlier, I would have lost her.

My wife is the perfect foil for me. The weaknesses in me seem to be her strongest points. This helps me find a greater balance in my life.

Synergy- two or more things working together to be more successful than the individual on its own. In my case that's is certainly true.

During my wedding speech I claim she was the shy and retiring type and that I was loud and outspoken. Anyone who knows us will know that I was the complete opposite.

I say "was" due to the fact I feel she has made me more confident in myself without me being on a high with bipolar to generate that feeling.

After only being together for 9 months, the decision to move into a flat together was a great move. I was then I started to grow as person, I had my first taste of independence and in control of proper grown up responsibilities, which was something I wouldn't think was possible years before.

Certainly, looking back to when I was spending all that time in hospital. Thinking that I was never going to get out, to get to the point where I was living independently and paying my own way through life felt amazing.

Chapter Twelve Proper routine

After I left the dream job of working with Kevin Keegan, I had asked my dad if he had any jobs going at his company.

That was supposed to be a short-term fix to get back in full time work.

Fast forward over ten years and I'm still at the same employment.

The company has been good for me in terms of making me more confident and a more grounded person.

I'm positive I would have been sacked in any other job for falling asleep at my desk due to high doses of medication. Or nights I had endless energy that my thoughts were racing well into the early hours of the next day, which lead me turning up the next day with huge bags under my eyes.

This lifestyle gave me the correct balance in which to stay stable all these years.

In 2015 I started voluntary work for Bi-Polar Scotland. This was a local self-help group. I was the chairperson for this group. While it was an eye opener to an extent, I feel like I would have been more suited to a sort of front-line role. A role where the person has just had a diagnosis, or where their family member is new to the situation.

I left that position in the weeks leading up to my first-born arriving. When things settle, I found out the group closed with the lack of numbers attending.

Chapter Thirteen

The dream

Picture the scene. I'm looking down at my hands holding a microphone. The curtains open and I'm faced with hundreds of eyes on me...

The noise is deafening as I reach the centre of then stage. The cheers die down and my story starts from a video behind me projected on a huge screen.

My life story plays out and then I narrate through the bipolar experience, recovery and the progression.

That's when I woke up in a hot sweat. I hate public speaking....

After talking to a room of around one hundred guests at my wedding and finding the heart to read a poem about my Grandma at her funeral makes me think maybe it could be possible one day.

The dream, the possibilities of talking about this very book and the reasons for doing it make me think that it could be a reality. The reality would most likely be in front of a small classroom but, shoot for the stars eh? Why not.

Chapter Fourteen

Starting a family

I thought that I had a good outlook and perspective on what life should be like.

All of that changed on a Monday night in July 2016.

Seeing the world through a parent's eye has brought a whole new ball into the game of life.

Throughout my childhood I had always been around kids through my forever extending family.

I love seeing a younger person grow up and enjoy watching how they develop.

In early Autumn 2019 my wife brought another ray of light into my life.

I hope the mistakes and lessons I have learnt can shape the way I will bring my children up in this world.

Hopefully those experiences that I went through gives me a major advantage on what advice to pass down towards them.

I hope they will gain a huge grasp of mental health and how important it is to be open and honest with others regarding it.

I know they must make their own mistakes, but I will always be around to support them and do my best to guide them.

I hope they will look up to their dad and be proud of what I am trying to do.

Chapter Fifteen

The time to start writing

Although I have laid pen to paper numerous times throughout the years trying to piece this story together. Nothing seemed to click before. I was missing the key link to put it all together.

Maybe the time just wasn't right, maybe I wasn't focused enough or maybe just maybe I have only now managed to express how I feel and why I had felt certain emotions times.

You might call it growing up, I grew up with this illness years ago. But to have confidence in my own skin to finally lay it all bare in front of my own eyes (and anyone else's) has taken me to new depths that I didn't think were possible.

I have had to stop numerous times during this process because I dived far too deep and had to think about my own health suffering again.

Reading Frank Bruno's "let me be Frank".

Franks story is quite remarkable.

The man must be truly admired for his grit and determination.

Reading his book "let me be Frank" gave me flashbacks to a lot of memories and made me realise it wasn't just me who felt all that emotion.

It's the only book I have managed to read from cover to cover and feel connected with it. Not once wanting to wander mid story.

Most books that I have ever bought I tend to not go the distance. I tend to get distracted from them and never go the full 12 rounds.

That book had me gripped. Mainly due to knowing his back story and wanting to find out how he coped.

He too felt betrayed. His active lifestyle like mine (in some sense) had to take a back seat. He too was sectioned and forced back into a corner. No bell would ring to take him out of that fight.

Grandma

One key role model in my life was my Grandma. She was well respected and stood up for what she believed in. She had that strict look, and whenever you saw it you knew you had done something wrong or had to toe the line. Being able to look at someone without ever laying a finger on them was an art form. She had mastered that over many years.

She believed in the underdog. And always backed that person, no-matter what.

For me to be hit with this illness I knew myself that I was the underdog. My Grandma believed in me. She had told me numerous times throughout the years. More so when it was just me and her together. Invariably, when I picked her up in my car to drive her about, in that moment she would tell me, not making eye contact but just looking straight ahead. I often wondered why at those moments she would tell me. I think it would probably be the time I was focused, and I would be listening.

It was my Grandma who taught me to tell the time. It's now my time to help others.

Chapter Sixteen

My thoughts

Mental illness

Your mental health is like a balloon with the knot tied.

Mental ill health is squeezing more air in. The more it takes in, with every squeeze, one day it's going to explode or deflate and buzz off into the atmosphere.

It can be prevented if you release some air. You need to learn how to do this.

It has taken me years to come to terms with it.

First, I had to come to terms with the fact that I have a mental health condition. I never wanted to believe I did.

Talking is the ideal solution for this, or just writing your thoughts down on paper. A physical injury can be diagnosed then fixed by someone else. Only the individual truly knows what thoughts are going on in their head, these thoughts need to be discussed.

Secondly to find the solution to help maintain a good state of mind, whether it be through a good routine or taking time to focus on yourself.

Chapter Seventeen

Doctors notes

"David shows signs of depression, I advise further time in the ward"

What a crock of shit that is! This is supposed to be a professional.

Who wouldn't feel down at being kept in hospital with no fresh air and being told you can't leave the building?

Doctors called it intrusive thoughts without explaining what they meant by saying it. A lot of medical jargon thrown around, and at the time sailed right over my head. Added to the fact the medication slowed my thought process down. Anything a doctor would say would take a while to grasp, and when I did realise what they were actually talking about I was out of the meeting, heartbroken in my room after being told I had to remain for another set amount of time.

I feel the doctors should have got a better understanding of me, not just through my close relates but also with my friends.

My friends would have been able to see things in a better perspective of how I live my life. And how I am when at ease.

The doctors tried me on 4 different medications before a mix of two different types finally worked for me.

1. Olanzapine

Olanzapine is an antipsychotic medication that affects chemicals in the brain. **Olanzapine** is used to treat the symptoms of psychotic conditions such as schizophrenia and bipolar disorder (manic depression) in adults and children who are at least 13 years old

Source – drugs.com

2. Lithium

Lithium compounds, also known as **lithium** salts, are primarily used as a psychiatric **medication**. This includes the treatment of major depressive disorder that does not improve following the use of other antidepressants, and bipolar disorder. In these disorders, it reduces the risk of suicide.

Source – Wikipedia

3. Amisulphrate

sold under the brand name Solian among others, is an antipsychotic medication used to treat schizophrenia. It is also used to treat dysthymia. It is usually classed with the atypical antipsychotics.

Source Wikipedia

4 Quetiapine

Quetiapine FUMARATE. ... This medication is used to treat certain mental/mood conditions (such as schizophrenia, bipolar disorder, sudden episodes of mania or depression associated with bipolar disorder). **Quetiapine** is known as an anti-psychotic drug (atypical type).

Source - webmd

5 Depakote and risperidone

Depakote (divalproex sodium) affects chemicals in the body that may be involved in causing seizures. ... Depakote is also used to treat manic episodes related to bipolar disorder (manic depression), and to prevent migraine headaches

Risperidone, sold under the brand name Risperdal among others, is an atypical antipsychotic. It is used to treat schizophrenia, bipolar disorder, and irritability associated with autism. It is taken either by mouth or by injection into a muscle. The injectable version is long-acting and lasts for about two weeks.

Source drugs.com and Wikipedia

Chapter Eighteen

Family thoughts

I asked these questions to my family who were present at the time.

1. What was your initial thoughts on my diagnosis?

2. Did you relate the illness with any behaviour as a kid?

3. Did you understand what the diagnosis meant? Did you go away and read up on it?

4. Were you worried about my long-term health?

5. Did you think I shouldn't have been in hospital at the times I was in?

6. How did you feel about the "mental hospital" tag on me?

7. Was there a point in my "illness" that could have been misrepresented by normal youth rebellion behaviour?

Dad

1. What was your initial thoughts on my diagnosis?

Mostly fear, worry and confusion. It was several weeks, months before we were eventually advised by the hospital Consultants that you had "bipolar." Several friends and family talked about Schizophrenia. Of having a split personality and all the theatrical images that this threw up. No one really described you as bipolar but referred a lot to manic depression. My early thoughts and hopes where that you had taken "something" and that you would eventually return to normal! All we wanted was our wee boy back!

2. Did you relate the illness with any behaviour as a kid?

No. You were always a quiet, shy, caring and loving child. I was always concerned that you were not outward enough but there was nothing in your behaviour that gave us any indication of what was about to happen.

3. Did you understand what the diagnosis meant? Did you go away and read up on it?

Initially no. Yes. we were told what the likely effects were. We were also told that you could have one episode in your life and or never another one for years to come. Our worst fears were when we were told that your illness was cyclical and was likely to re-occur rapidly.

I spent days, weeks and months, reading health articles in journals and books, on health authority websites and on google searches, looking for an answer or a "cure". Some articles gave me hope whilst others shattered any illusions of "normality".

4. Were you worried about my long-term health?

Extremely worried. Once we knew what the illness was and how you were reacting to it, we knew that we were in for the long haul. We were of course hopeful that after the first episode and with the correct medication you would be fine, but we were to quickly learn that this illness was not going away. Mum and I had numerous conversations with your CPNs most of whom were hopeless apart from Scott Little, who by the time he came on the scene we were becoming more knowledgeable about the illness. When you were at home and out at your work or with your friends I constantly worried about you, wondering if you were ok and hoping that you had not harmed yourself or bought something expensive like a new car or a holiday. You were never sleeping during your manic episodes and tearful and withdrawn during your depressed state. During that period, I worried about your future, in education, in work, in marriage and in fatherhood. I honestly thought at that time that there would be no more grandchildren and if there was, would they be bipolar as well!

5. Did you think I shouldn't have been in hospital at the times I was in?

When you first presented your manic side on my return from England on the 3rd February, there was no doubt in my mind that you were seriously ill. Granma had phoned to say that you had said that I allowed you and your mates to take alcohol from the drinks cabinet and I put that down to teenage exuberance. Little did I know what was about to explode within the next few days. On the 4th of February I have never felt as hopeless, helpless and terrified, as we went from the house to the GP and subsequently to the "mad house." Dykebar hospital was familiar to me through my professional life as I had to serve Curator Bonis petitions on mentally in patients in locked wards. I thought that you would see a doctor, be given medication and come home with me later once the meds had kicked in. Dykebar was an old Victorian Hospital, which has admitted by the healthcare authorities was not suitable for keeping young people in but since there was no other place available and given how ill you were, there was no choice. We were at the mercy of the professionals and although we were extremely upset about it, on the first occasion we had no choice. Neither did we have a choice on the occasions you were sectioned but we visited every day, most of the time with my shiny shoes on, and constantly continued with our dialogue with consultants, the legal agents and mental health organisations. We were told on numerous occasions that our frequent visits were not helping and that we should cut down the time we spent with you, as it was felt that this would eventually stop you from getting over anxious and sometimes aggressive when we did. This was a very difficult concept to accept.

I think that you should have been hospitalised on each occasion but not necessarily sectioned or detained for the period that you were. Particularly the time that you spent in Gartnavel.

6. How did you feel about the "mental hospital" tag on me?

Initially, I think everyone thought "what must people be thinking" Oh! how embarrassing having a son in the "nut house." You and we were no doubt the talk of the town, but our thoughts quickly turned to you and how you would be affected. It was so hard but so brave of you going back to school, personally I don't think I could have done it. You also faced up to life, strongly and resolutely during those 5 years of trying to be "normal" whilst working with the knowledge that this was going to be a lifetime struggle. Your Mum and I desperately struggled with our shared thoughts, often bursting into tears, worrying about you and your future. Eventually the "tag" faded and became unimportant. Even during those lost 5 years you showed strength and endurance and a determination to prove that you would not be beaten. You have used the "tag" to your advantage to show everyone that mental health illness can affect anyone, and it is through you that the world is beginning to accept and embrace this fact.

7. Was there a point in my "illness" that could have been misrepresented by normal youth rebellion behaviour?

Sorry but no. I only wish that it had. Certainly, on the 4th February my explanation of your strange behaviour was that you had obviously taken "something" but was soon to realise that the effects of Cannabis do not last for 5 years.

Feel free to add in any other points.

As a father my only regrets are what we missed doing during those 5 lost years. Going to the pub, the football and just doing generally what fathers and sons do during the teenage and adolescence years.

I have watched you grow into a remarkable, caring and loving husband and father. Yes, you missed out on university and many other teenage opportunities but the education of life which you have had, is in my opinion, made you what you are today.

As I said to you earlier, there are many more thoughts which your Mum, Lynne, myself and even Laura could add to this courageous auto biography but perhaps we should leave them to be included in the second novel.

Mum

1. What was your initial thoughts on my diagnosis?

At the beginning I hadn't a clue what was happening having never come across anything like this. After being told what it might be. I went and looked online and that made it even more confusing.

> 2. *Did you relate the illness with any behaviour as a kid?*

Not at all. You were always very quiet as a child apart from when you were annoying Laura. If we went out anywhere you hardly said a word.

> 3. *Did you understand what the diagnosis meant? Did you go away and read up on it?*

No, I didn't understand what was wrong as at the beginning they weren't sure either. They thought you had an episode of some sort. One minute you were high then low. Reading up on it made me feel worse wondering what else was to come

> 4. *Were you worried about my long-term health?*

Yes. I thought he would get medication and that would fix him. As time went on and with different medication nothing changed. Visiting every afternoon and evening was very draining. When they put you on Lithium, we thought it would help but with your fear of needles having to get blood tests all the time you were getting more stressed, so they took you off that.

> 5. *Did you think I shouldn't have been in hospital at the times I was in?*

I didn't think you should have been in Dykebar at the beginning as you were only 16 and everyone in there were much older.

When you went into the Adolescent unit, I thought it was a much better place for you with people your own age.

> 6. *How did you feel about the "mental hospital" tag on me?*

At the time I never thought about that just wanted to get you better and out of those places and back to you leading a normal life.

> 7. *Was there a point in my "illness" that could have been misrepresented by normal youth rebellion behaviour?*

No, I don't think so. You had always been a quiet child and never been any trouble so when you started acting strangely, we knew something wasn't right.

Feel free to add in any other points.

Just wanted to say how proud I am off how you are now after everything you have been through and how Karen has helped you and of course my two Beautiful Grandchildren Neave and Ben. Love you. Mum xx

Sister

At the time of the initial onset of David's illness, I had been living away from home for a few years in Milton Keynes after going travelling. Over the course of a couple of weeks my mum had spoken to me on the phone, voicing her concerns about David's behaviour. David had always been a 'good boy' but had split up from his first serious girlfriend and was taking it quite badly. His strange behaviour was out of character and had caused the teachers to suspect he was using drugs.

There had been a couple on minor incidents and David's relationship with my dad seemed to be deteriorating. This could have been put down to 'normal' teenage rebellion, but it all came to a head in February 2002 when I got a phone call at work. My mum was crying and all I could hear was my Dad and David screaming and fighting in the background. It felt like this call went on for hours, but it was probably only a few minutes until the police arrived. I felt completely helpless being miles away and my initial instinct was to jump in the car and drive home - but I wasn't sure what I could do to help.

The next few days were a bit of a blur and it felt like the doctors didn't really know what was wrong. David was sectioned and there was talk of drugs and schizophrenia. Mum and Dad were mentally and physically bruised but also feeling guilty as to whether there was anything they could/ should have done differently. Combined with my sister's Down Syndrome and me now living 350 miles away, they felt like they were being punished for something. I felt guilty too, thinking maybe if I hadn't moved away, he may have confided in me about how he was feeling and maybe prevented him being sectioned.

I eventually decided to drive up and see David for myself rather than hearing second hand. I remember nervously entering the hospital and really wasn't sure what to expect. I almost didn't recognise him - it was like a different version of my brother. He'd lost a lot of weight and was clearly agitated. At times he was quite hostile to my dad and seemed to hold him responsible for the situation.

His behaviour varied wildly from day to day and I wasn't sure how much was down to the drugs they were administering or whether it was his illness. Sometimes it was like someone had sucked all the life and energy from David. His eyes were glazed, he wasn't washing, and he seemed like he had given up. At other times, he became like an artist, channelling his creativity to write poetry, songs and doing drawings. He talked constantly and described scenarios and situations which we knew had never happened or were never going to happen.

Eventually the doctors started discussing an illness called bipolar disorder. It wasn't something that I had ever heard of, but it certainly sounded less scary than schizophrenia. I immediately started reading up on it to understand more. Manic depression was mentioned in most articles which was a more familiar term. I could understand the depression side to the illness, but the descriptions of the manic episodes were scary.

With hindsight, we can now laugh at some of the things David did during his manic episodes, but these are what concerned me most, in terms of affecting his long-term future – both in his career and financially. He would go on spending sprees - booking holidays, buying cars and even went to the Rangers football ground, convinced that he had a trial. He later downgraded his expectations and went to St Mirren instead, which still makes me chuckle! My dad spent a lot of time trying to reverse the purchases and commitments that David had made using all his legal knowledge and local networks to overturn these.

Despite how poorly David was during his periods in hospital, I wasn't overly worried about his long-term health. I'm an optimist anyway (or perhaps naive) but everything I read suggested that the illness was treatable.

With regards the stigma of a 'mental health' label, this wasn't immediately a concern of mine. To me, David was just ill, whether it was mental or physical illness, didn't really matter. It was only when he was moved to a hospital called 'Dykebar', that it hit home a bit more. This hospital was the place that we joked about as kids as the place where the 'nutters' go. I could imagine David's peers talking and joking about it, and it worried me how he might be treated when/ if he went back to school.

In 2020, the stigma of mental health is reducing but there is still a long way to go, especially for men. Hopefully this book can help to increase awareness and open people's eyes to the reality of living with mental illness – not just for those with the mental illness, but also their friends and family. It also shows that there is light at the end of the tunnel, despite how long and dark that tunnel can seem at the start.

Chapter Nineteen

The St Andrews day interview 2017

On November 30th, 2017 I had a skype interview with a researcher from Manchester University.

It was the first time I felt like I could really open to a stranger.

The interview came about after answering a post that "Bi-polar Scotland" had put online.

"To interview twelve people who have had a diagnosis of any bipolar disorder. To ask them about their experiences of working towards being able to live the life they want."

The interview was done in two one-hour slots over a couple of weeks.

Whilst being interviewed I felt completely at ease and could describe everything I felt at each point in time. As the questions moved deeper into the condition, I could feel myself holding up that same guard I always held up. You know that guard you hold up when someone asks you how you are and your go to response is always "fine".

Well, she was able to smash through that guard, I had only ever let people close to me in until that point.

I relaxed and got deeper into the conversation. Her leading questions started to open my memories and it became a lot easier to discuss the things that happened to me over those key years.

She went on to interview another 9 people and some of the findings were very similar to my experiences.

The study was as follows:

"We wanted to further understand what people once diagnosed with bipolar disorders felt was important in them changing their life to make it more the way they wanted it to be. We hope that increasing our understanding of what is involved will help shift current negative attitudes and assumptions about the long-term nature of this diagnosis"

The keys things that I feel matched my thoughts with other people are:

1. Acknowledging that there was a problem which was described as a turning point for many. It allows access to treatment and further support.

2. Everyone showed a willingness of trial and error of medication until something worked.

3. Everyone had taken medication. The majority still take medication today.

4. Following recognising the problem, people had an instinctive curiosity in then finding out more about the diagnosis. People said that they wanted to learn more about bipolar disorder and knowhow to manage it. Some people read about how others with the diagnosis had made changes. Many people wanted to help others now by talking about what they had found helpful about bipolar disorder and things like that

5. Taking control of your own lives was important. People started to feel more in charge of their recovery.

6. Changing how I think included thinking about what things were like in the past. Looking back to see the progress we had made. It helps to identify dark thoughts.

7. Accepting who I am and how I feel.

8. The largest category was described as looking after me. This included people understanding themselves more and how bipolar disorder affected them. They identified what things made them feel worse. People started to do more things that they loved and prioritised their own needs more. These things helped them feel and stay well.

Upon looking at those findings from the interview I took part it. It started to give me a greater sense of not being alone with bipolar. Something that I really struggled with at the beginning.

Chapter Twenty

The penultimate hope

The aim of the putting these open and honest feelings laid to paper is to try and help anyone effected in the way I was. As the old cliché goes, if one person can take inspiration from my story then I will be pleased.

I hope my experiences will help the kids of today. The teenagers that going through that change of life, who are trying to find who they are in this world.

To the adults who haven't managed to understand and grasp the demons that have been locked inside all these years.

And in general, to provide knowledge of Bi-polar and mental health as a whole and try and eliminate the stigma that comes with it.

I hope the recurring nightmares I have about waking up in a psychiatric ward never happen to anyone else.

The final chapter

The conclusion.

I have spent over two years creating this book. Starting from St Andrews day 2017. While piecing together the story of my bipolar years, I managed to obtain my doctors notes. These helped me recall memories and situations I found myself under. Those memories were moments that crushed me at the time. These are the times I felt powerless and mentally boxed in a corner.

How I went from an outwardly shy boy to a grown adult.

The key points of my story which I tried to get across were these:

• Being diagnosed with bipolar at the age of 16. With no understanding of mental health conditions.

• Having four sectioned hospital admissions and one voluntary stay which ended up as a section.

• Extreme highs with psychosis and an endless supply of energy.

• Extreme lows with feelings of worthlessness.

• How playing football helped me come out of my depressive state after my final stay in hospital.

• Staying with that football peer group helped build up social skills and confidence.

• How the importance of a balanced lifestyle with rest and a decent amount of physical activity.

- How important it is to take ownership (the realisation step) of your own mental health and seek professional help.

The disorder

Looking back over my early years I could see stages of bipolar. Days of full energy and days with no energy. Some reckless thoughts and daydreams. Some nights where I wouldn't go to sleep until very late/early morning.

I was sectioned three times before my 18th birthday. Maybe the fact that I was so young and slightly naïve enhanced those episodes occurring more frequently.

Possibly the notion of wanting to feel high again wouldn't have mattered what age I was at the time.

I have been asked before "if you could take a magic pill and bipolar will disappear would you take it?"

My answer is no! I believe it was meant to play out the way it did.

I firmly think I would be a different person today if I didn't go through it all. It has opened my eyes up to whole new side of life, to things I never thought possible. It has given me a clearer picture of what is important and what I should stress about.

Everything I have experienced has shaped the way I think today. To feel more empathy for people than I already did. To not look down on anyone and see the best in them.

The experience of the "high" is something I will never forget. The sense of greatness, over self-confidence, high energy, and rapid thoughts.

In all honesty I miss feeling like that. I mean who wouldn't want to feel great about themselves all the time?

The "high" was the main reason I ended back up in hospital a few times. I had stopped taking medication because I wanted to feel like that again.

I have always wondered about the person you become with a Bi-polar high. Is this the reflection of the person you wish you really were?

This was the situation that I couldn't grasp. When in the cusp of an elevated state, how could I be ill when I felt so good?

However, when you are that high ultimately there is only one way you can go. And that's down. That's the opposite effect. The longer I was high the more of a crash I got. The fall back down to earth. The flip side to bi-polar was the depression.

The great depression, the ones with no self-confidence, no energy and dark thoughts. Feelings of worthlessness.

A blank mind staring up at the ceiling. No focus. No drive. Nothing!

Things that stress people in day to day life doesn't bother me, because I know there is a much harder place I could be. I'm lucky I managed to get though all the episodes in good shape. I am almost horizontal now when it comes to dealing with stress.

The bi-polar state of mind will always be in the back on my head though.

Sometimes I wonder if today is the day when it starts to bite back.

However, it will take a momentous situation for me ever to go backwards.

With the help of years practicing good health and recognising my triggers has made my life easier. Together with the good support network I have around me.

I have memorised the a4 sheet of paper I worked on with my CPN.

This A4 sheet split in two columns highlighted early warning signs and things to do to get help.

I have promised myself that I would catch whatever gets thrown at me. And never let anything fester inside me.

My normal/rational thoughts may vary with whatever life throws at me.

Trying to block out mental ill health will never happen. I can forget about it in the course of the day by being busy but at night it's the routine medication that keeps me focused.

Some nights my mind is going faster than it should when trying to wind down, but that is dependent on the day I have had.

Hospital life

Looking back to times where I was isolated a room to myself with nothing but my own thoughts. That's just a mind fuck. These times when I was at my extreme high. Instead of leaving my mind to its own devices, my mind should have been stimulated then gradually wound down.

On the other hand, bi-polar affects people in many ways. Doctors action plan's must be tailor made on each individual person.

However, if gave the doctors all my thoughts, they would literally have been blown out the stratosphere.

I used to always wonder how I was supposed to act in an environment where everything you do is written down or relayed for some else to interpret. Do you act like you are happy to stay in this environment? Should you be content with the situation you are in, locked up in unit against your wishes?

On occasions I would get day trips where I would go home and visit my friends. Sometimes after weeks spent away from them. After longer weeks apart it was more difficult to adjust to seeing them again. Sometimes I wouldn't recognise them due to hair growth.

After spending copious amounts of time in hospital the feeling of being institutionalised was very real. I feared going home. Being home was the only place I had felt safe. But now I was scared going places, interacting with people outside the unit and that made me feel about two feet tall.

Education

To start with. I missed out on getting my qualifications and going to university. I thought that was the benchmark at the time and something I must achieve.

The social side of uni ended up being no issue as my friends would invite me to the events they went to. On these occasions I would invent up some wild stories to strangers who asked me what course I was on.

But back then that's what I wanted. It's what I thought I should be doing with my life.

All my mates were at Uni and I was in and out a fucking mental hospital!

Exercise

Keeping active has been a vital part of keeping a lid on my mental health. From going for hill sprints at 10pm to playing football regularly and going long walks with my family.

Medication

I drew up a list on the doctor's notes part of the different medications I have taken. I am currently I am on the lowest dose of Depakote. I am still holding on to the fact it works for me and wouldn't want to part from it. Well not just yet.

Current climate

I have often wondered what it would be like if I was that skinny 16-year-old today. Would social media play a major role in my situation?

Would my meltdown have went viral? Would I have suffered from people trolling me about my mental health?

Back then we only had dial up internet connection at home and snake on our Nokia 3210's!

Right now, it would be a harder to deal with it what I went through?

I know stigma is on the decrease in society, but that doesn't stop kids being kids and indirectly damaging someone else's character. Such as making fun of them to make themselves look good around other kids.

Although in 2020, a lot of mental health issues are being spoken about. But people are still throwing phrases like he's having a bi-polar day around the office. Going on my experience alone.

Motivation

I have always been motivated to keep going forward. Even during the times when I struggled and felt I was never going to get out hospital in the short term. In my head this was never going to be the path I was going to stay on.

Proving the doubters wrong.

After all the negative comments to my face, or more times than not, behind my back. I always prove that those comments a generally unfounded. It gives me great pleasure in facing up to these challenges which are thrown in my way.

The setbacks I make and the mistakes I learn from and help me grow going forward.

Tackling stigma

However, times are changing! More and more mental health charities are coming to the fore front.

Brilliant set ups such as Aaron Connelly's Time to tackle initiative. This joint group set up with his wife gives participants an hour of football. Followed by a relaxed environment to chat and be supported from within the group.

Furthermore, this group has expanded and holds charity days in conjunction with other charities which have the same ideas.

This type of initiative would have helped me immensely at the time. Playing football, keeping fit, and surrounded in a supportive peer group.

Mental health stigma is slowing being eliminated. More and more men and women are speaking up about Mental Health issues in the public eye and I couldn't be happier.

Final statement

I used to look over my shoulder to see if bipolar was going to attack me. Right now, I have a firm grasp of it in front of me, held tightly in my own hands.

I know that it will be a constant battle and that I will never stopping going toe to toe with it. I won't turn my back on it. However, I might need to lean on the ropes(support) if I must have that inch of space.

I am prepared to fight. It will never be time to take those gloves off or throw in the towel.

My bi-polar story will never finish, this fight-back has been for that skinny 16-year-old kid back on the Fourth of February 2002.

From being stuck in the darkness to emerging into the bright lights of hope.

Printed in Great Britain
by Amazon